STRESS, WE ARE DONE

STRESS, WE ARE DONE

Practical Strategies To Manage Any Stress And Work Consistently At Peak Performance Without Breaking Down, Including Relatable Stories From Real People.

EZINNE M. NNAMDI-LOUIS MD

DEDICATION

This book is dedicated to all high performing individuals who are working hard to make the world a better place, through their various skills and competences. Also to my dearest husband, Nnamdi Louis Okeke, and beloved daughter, Kosi, who are my perfect gifts in this stress management journey.

FOREWORD

As a physician-cum-entrepreneur, I have seen and experienced the effects of stress. I have also witnessed adverse effects of prolonged and unmanaged stress. They are everywhere around us, often overlooked and frequently misunderstood.

This is why I appreciate the wealth of information contained in this book and the impact it made in my life. I am not surprised at how meticulous the research was, considering I have known Dr. Ezinne Nnamdi-Louis for several years and have seen firsthand her dedication and passion for people.

STRESS WE ARE DONE, explains in simple and easily understood terms, the daily battle between stress and the average man; from the hardworking breadwinner to the high-flying executive. You will not find any medical jargon here, this book was written to be understood and it's information implemented by all. There are also real-life stories of people who were faced with certain stressful situations and how they overcame; real lessons to us all. STRESS WE ARE DONE, will answer all your questions on stress and I urge you to read and practice all you will learn from this awesome book.

-Dr. Marvellous Njoku

Founder, PURE SUCCESS PRO

INTRODUCTION

Not long ago, I had an interesting conversation with my mum. She had attended the August meeting and given a lecture on stress management. August meeting involves the annual gathering of women from the same region in August. It is common in the eastern part of Nigeria.

I was surprised, I wondered what she had taught them on the topic. She explained that she told them about taking things easy and not losing themselves as they work hard to fend for their families. She spoke from experience because, in addition to her job as a teacher, she ran a full-scale business that flourished. Some knowledge I know about business is from her. She didn't attend a business school neither did she read books on business but her model is part of what we learn in books today. Needless to say, she is very wise and hardworking too.

Back to her teachings during the August meeting; she gave illustrations, including a lady that lost her life very early to stress. Then she said to me, "If I had read your teachings on Stress Management, I would have told them more".

That was one of the proudest moments of my life.

When she was done, I tried to give her a mini-lecture on stress management to further equip her as an advocate. I began by telling her how stress is the body's natural response to a perceived threat or a huge demand and how the body responds with slight increases in blood pressure, heart rate, and respiration.

However, she cut me short that she wasn't interested in such details.

That was when it dawned on me that to effectively communicate with my audience, I had to go straight to the language they will understand and not just talk about some scientific findings.

From her discussion at the women's meeting, it was clear that she delivered the message better because she used real-life situations to convey the message. I have observed that the middle-aged and the elderly advocate about stress management greatly because they have witnessed the life and they know better now.

So, in this book, you are not going to encounter some medical or scientific jargon. No. You will be reading true stories from real people who have overcome various life stresses. The aim is to impact you with information that you would always remember to practice daily.

By the time you finish reading this book, you will be more equipped to cope with any form of life stress without losing your sanity or life.

In all your ventures, don't let stress cut short your lifespan.

Table of Contents

SECTION 1

IT IS NOT YOUR FAULT

CHAPTER 1

Can We Be Done With Stress?

S ometimes when I talk about the importance of managing stress, there is a set of people that don't seem to understand me. People who are not interested in any extra effort, who don't care so much about where they are going or interested in any responsibilities. They do not understand, because with a sense of responsibility, comes stress.

In other words, to avoid stress, you either become a newborn or exit the world. This means that as long as we exist on this earth, we are going to experience different degrees of stress.

The young adult is stressed about school and sometimes, how to make money while the older ones are worried about meeting the ever-increasing daily needs. The married are worried about intermittent marital conflicts, raising children, and supporting their future. The employer and employee are worried about stress at work. The priest/pastor is worried about his congregation's welfare, and so on.

This reminds me of the days my mum read the bible to me as a child. One verse by Solomon stuck, "the wiser you are, the more worries you have"

These words are so true.

You see, you feel stressed because you care; because you are wise; because you want a change; because you want a better life.

That means it will be unfair to beat yourself up for how you feel. It is simply your body responding to a situation and telling you to do something about it. It is not your fault.

You may ask; "If stress is not my fault, why then do I have to learn to manage it?" The reason is, even though it is your body's natural response, the problem arises when you don't do anything about the situation or when you handle the situation wrongly.

We will discuss more on this in the next section.

As I write this, I'm in the hospital because my child is here for observation. It's about midnight and it's costing me my sleep. I could have chosen to ignore whatever was going on and selfishly "live my best life", but I chose this responsibility because I want the best for her.

Choosing to be responsible is not only for parents. It is also for the man or woman who wants to make an impact and share his/her gifts/ talents with the world. It is for people who want to live and not just exist; the company CEOs, the young entrepreneurs, the employees, the ministers, etc. and everyone who is making the world a better place to live in.

If you are in this category, I must commend you for being a world-changer; from the effort you put into making an impact in your family as the best husband, wife or child, to the creation of some innovative solutions to the problems of mankind. You could have chosen not to care about humanity but you decided otherwise. You are doing great and I applaud you.

However, as long as you have chosen to be responsible in life, you are going to encounter stress in various forms and if not handled, this exposure to high levels of stress will cost you in the long run.

I am not here to blame you for being responsible, quite the opposite. I want you to know that you can have it all, and that you can fulfill your dreams AND be in good health to enjoy it.

Unlike the man who doesn't care so much, yet suffers consequences of inaction later in life, you will learn some valuable life hacks that will help you navigate through the stresses of the journey and still come out healthier, good-looking and strong enough to reap the fruit of your labors.

As a doctor, I have witnessed patients who have come in with stroke due to uncontrolled high blood pressure and other related diseases, and who eventually lost their lives. Some of these patients were people's parents who worked daily to cater for their families.

You cannot blame them for choosing to take care of their homes because that is what every responsible person would do, however, many people get lost in what should be done that they neglect to also take care of themselves. This is usually due to ignorance.

For instance, a man in his 50s who is a driver would always leave the house early in the morning for work. By the time he gets home, he is exhausted. There are bills to pay and if he misses work any day, he gets no money for that day. He may be experiencing recurrent headaches and dizziness, but because of the numerous bills, he sees going to the hospital as a luxury. He would rather go to a nearby pharmacy and drown in regular painkillers.

Does this sound like anyone you know? Very likely.

Unfortunately, he doesn't recognize, neither is he aware of what stress is and how it affects the body. Furthermore, he may not know that he suffers high blood pressure, which is being worsened by the stress. Next, he is rushed to the hospital because he fell while having his bath, and a diagnosis of stroke is made by the doctors.

The story you just read is not to scare you but to make you understand the realities people face when they choose to be responsible in life. Sadly, we are losing more industrious people to stress-related ailments.

The good news is that this will never be your story because you got this book, which will educate you and prepare you to live a healthier life. This is why you must practice whatever you learn from this book, as a lifestyle. I strongly believe that if you do this, you will last longer in your service to humanity, in good health.

SECTION 2

BE AWARE

CHAPTER 3

Recognize The Warning Signs

Now that you are here, I assume that you have some ideas or none at all about the many dangers of stress. I'll make them clear to you as much as possible. Over the years I began this journey of stress management, I've asked one question over and over again. How do you recognize when your body is screaming, "I'm stressed?"

Pause and think.

While many tell me, "I feel headache", others complain of dizziness, body aches, confusion, or feeling frustrated, and irritable. I'm not surprised that most people don't know the warning signs their bodies give them until it gets too late, because of the low awareness regarding stress.

Imagine a rubber band. When you just throw it, it lands after a very short distance. But if you stretch it, it can propel further to a farther distance. However, if you continue stretching it, it will get to a point where it can't withstand the pressure and snaps.

This describes stress. It is not all bad, stress can also be useful.

To launch into greater heights, you will encounter various kinds of situations that will stress you. They could be negative or positive pressure. Your ability to understand when you have reached the limit your body can handle will determine whether the workload will break you or not.

That is what this chapter is about. It will help you recognize warning signs of too much stress, peculiar to your own body.

What are the benefits of knowing these warning signs?
- To increase your self-awareness and help you recognize quickly any negative stress signals.
- To avoid dire consequences of stress overload that will affect your health, productivity, and happiness.
- To help you maximize your productivity. This is because we are all wired differently by genetic makeup, environmental influence, underlying health condition, etc. and understanding how your body works will benefit you.

What this means is that our bodies warn us in different ways, which is why you should not rely on Mr. B's interpretation of his body's cues, even when you two are doing the same job.

Relate it to morning and night workers. A person who usually has more energy in the morning will do less in the evenings and vice versa because of the understanding they have of their bodies and when best they work at peak performance.

In the same vein, if you get signals to rest after 4 hours of work, it will be counterproductive to keep working because your productivity will reduce. That is why some people will boast of sleeping only 5 hours and achieve results, while you will need 7 hours of sleep to achieve the same.

In essence, be self-aware and understand your body perfectly.

I had a client who complained of recurrent chest vibrations. He went in and out of the hospital several times until a doctor explained to him that stress was the trigger. When I talked to him, we observed a trend. The symptoms came on towards evening (after work hours) and went away by morning (after a good night's rest). So, we mapped out strategies to cut down the stress at work and it worked.

I have had another client who spent so much in the hospital looking for a particular cause of her problem. It got worse that she thought someone was after her life.

Do you see how it degenerated to a mental health issue?

After consultations with a psychiatrist, she discovered that a stressful life event was the trigger. These true-life instances further show you the need to know the warning signs of stress.

In my online community, I tell them; Stress can get you fired.

Imagine that you are working in a very reputable company and you have been asked to represent the company in promoting a product that will boost their income. Because you are stressed by the frustration of your toxic boss, you have lost your sleep and are now experiencing forgetfulness.

What do you think will be the outcome of that presentation? Of course, disaster.

Tony (not his real name) had a driver at his workplace. On one occasion, he gave the driver some instructions and to his surprise, the driver shouted at him. Tony, being an understanding man, realized that there must have been a fundamental issue because that was not the driver's usual attitude. He ignored the event to attend to more pressing issues.

Later that day, Tony called the now-apologetic driver and asked for an explanation for the outburst. The driver (let's call him Ade) calmly explained about how frustrated he was in a company that didn't care about his welfare.

He had called in sick, but he was threatened that his pay will be reduced if he missed any day at work. That led to his frustration. Had Tony not been an understanding boss, Ade could have been fired immediately. This is not to excuse the company's unfairness.

Do you also know that stress is one major cause of negative habits?

I once had a conversation with a reputable man that traveled with me from Qatar to Nigeria about a year ago. After mentioning what I do as a stress management specialist, he began telling me about how he became addicted to smoking.

His kind of job is a very tedious one. Because of the stress, he and his friends began hanging out in the bar to smoke in other to "relieve the stress for the day". As they continued this routine, he realized that he began smoking even on less stressed days and that was how he became addicted.

Several high achievers rely heavily on coffee (due to the caffeine content) as their energy booster to cope with the increasing work demand. Others resort to alcohol drinking. While these will give you a heightened sense of calm, the long term effect is deleterious. These habits don't manage the stress, rather they mask the intense yearnings of your body to get rest or do something healthy to cope with the situation.

This partly explains why we are losing more hardworking people to the consequences of these negative coping habits.

Do you know that stress is recognized as a cause of divorce, child abuse, and reduced immunity (Your body's ability to fight diseases)?

I believe you now get the point on why it is very important to recognize warning signs of stress before it can cost you your health, happiness, productivity, income, and ultimately your life.

Exercise: Before you continue reading, pause, and write out 3 common warning signs your body gives you when you are stressed. Now you are done, go through the list below to identify any other subtle warnings you might have missed.

Below are over 40 signs of stress:

Poor memory

Poor judgment/decision making

Difficulty concentrating on a task

Reduced interest in things that usually interest you

Mental restlessness

Constant worrying

Forgetfulness

Focusing only on the negatives

Low self-esteem

Complaints by others about how your work is affecting your relationship with them

Reduced focus on things that matter

Poor coordination

Aggressiveness/unnecessary nagging

Irritability

Addiction to drugs/alcohol/smoking

Sleep problems

Eating problems with weight gain or weight loss.

Procrastination

Indecisiveness

Struggling to do something creative that you used to do easily.

Being withdrawn from people/poor attitude to people and work

Nervous habits like nail biting

Change in facial expression

Loss of sex drive

Feeling overwhelmed

Fear

Anxiety

Agitation

Moodiness

Loneliness

Frustration

Depression

Headache

Chest pain

Diarrhea

Tummy pain

Delayed/Absent menstruation

Worsening blood pressure

Worsening pimples

Fast aging process

Constant tiredness

Heart racing

Increased risk of stroke and heart diseases (including heart attack)

Reduced immunity causing frequent colds

Difficulty managing diabetes and other underlying medical conditions

SECTION 3

HOW TO MANAGE STRESS

CHAPTER 4

How To Manage Any Stress

W hen you encounter a stressful situation, ask yourself these questions; Why is this happening?; What can I do to stop me from feeling this way now?; How do I solve the situation moving forward?

FIRST QUESTION: WHY IS THIS HAPPENING?

You can only answer this if you are sufficiently self-aware to recognize when something is off. It may be recurrent headaches or body aches. We discussed this extensively in the previous chapter.

Note that this is not the time to tell yourself off with negative thoughts such as; I'm not good enough, my life is such a mess, I just have bad luck, etc.

Such negative thoughts will only lead to the following;

You will feel more terrible

Your mind will magnify the situation to make you feel worse. You will feel like you have lost total control of the situation (even if it is a small issue)

You will not have the necessary clarity to think about the solution

Remember our discussion in the first section. You feel this way because you are responsible. This will help you have the clarity to identify the root cause of the issue. We will address identifying root causes or triggers later.

SECOND QUESTION: WHAT CAN I DO TO STOP ME FROM FEELING THIS WAY NOW?

Is your body telling you to rest or could it be that it is telling you to get a job done? You know that moment when you have a target with the deadline approaching and your heart starts beating faster, making sleep difficult?

That is good stress, where you are reminded that there's a job that you need to get done. This kind of stress lasts for only a short while, and you will get relaxed after the job is done. However, it becomes a problem if you ignore the warning, probably because;

You do not understand what is going on.

You are repeatedly under the same situation (always not meeting your target).

You respond to it negatively; such as taking alcohol or other substances to relax.

In response to the question, the answer may be; "find a solution or get the job done", depending on the situation.

THIRD QUESTION: HOW DO I SOLVE THE SITUATION?

At this point, you are more clear-headed in finding the solution. It may mean;

1. **Avoid the trigger completely**: You can implement this in certain cases such as a toxic relationship or when an account you follow on social media is the cause of your stress.

2. **Actively work towards a change of situation**: For instance, if your work colleague is always troubling you, you calmly speak up. Note that I used the word, "calmly" because if you do otherwise, you are only going to worsen the situation. Another instance may involve looking for an alternative source of income to help you meet up with financial demands, in cases of financial stress.

3. **Remind yourself that the situation won't last long**: This was my workplace a few years ago. You know that kind of job where you already have anxiety going to work every morning because you don't know what will happen. I spent most of my day complaining along with my colleagues. As we did, I kept feeling worse about the job because as I focused on the errors of the workplace, I saw more problems. Unfortunately, I couldn't quit and at the same time, I couldn't speak up to the authorities due to the nature of the job. In that situation, I had to remind myself that it was temporary and stopped complaining. This helped me to start seeing the job in a different light. In other words, changing your perspective is a game-changer in managing any stress that you can't avoid or do anything about.

4. **Accept that there's absolutely nothing you can do about it and moving on with your life**: Have you experienced that unexpected break-up that left you shattered? That type that you know is irredeemable. Or you may have experienced a terrible loss. The way you feel after these kinds of events are not explainable because they are awful. These are situations where truly, there's nothing you can do to remedy it apart from giving yourself time to accept what has happened and moving on with your life. I have been in one such situations and I must agree with you that it is not easy to move on just like that. I'm not asking you to do so quickly.

Give yourself the much needed time, but remind yourself to move on once you are ready. I'm cheering you on.

CHAPTER 5

Unique Strategies To Handle Any Form Of Stress

BE INTENTIONAL IN PRACTICING GRATITUDE

Not long ago, I got a mail that I had greatly anticipated. With trembling hands, I opened it. To my utmost dismay, I saw the text boldly written...FAIL.
I failed an exam.

I didn't know how to take the news as I wasn't prepared for what I saw. Yes, I was among the high fliers in my class back then and wasn't used to failing an exam but this one happened.

Yes, I had thoughts like, "my life is over", "my career is gone", and "I'm finished". But I refused to utter them with my mouth. I worried about the time devoted to studying, money spent or rather wasted, energy consumed, etc.

While my mind was clouded by worries, I saw no reason to forge on. However, all of that changed when I remembered my wins that year, especially the previous month.

You see, I am a stress management coach, and countless times I have seen the amazing effect of intentionally practicing gratitude. Because I was intentional in recording my wins and God's blessings in the past, it was easy for me to recognize that I've had more wins than losses. This loss seemed major but it was not enough to make me ignorant of things that worked out.

I was also able to think clearly on how to forge ahead despite the failure. I was able to see opportunities to do better with my career. It wasn't easy within the first few hours I saw that mail but the path eventually seemed clearer on the next step to take.

It is usually our first instinct to whine about our failures and other stressors, and quickly forget the times we got it right. These disturbing situations can steal our peace of mind for a long time, depending on how much we allow it to.

"If you want to stay ahead of the unpleasant seasons of life, you must make gratitude a lifestyle"

Do this exercise:

Get a book of blessings (a journal or any exercise book).
Record every win and blessing you have experienced.

Note that this exercise may seem too insignificant and easily ignored, but I challenge you to do it consistently for a week, then a month, and eventually a year.

This is what will happen when you do so; when you feel like dwelling on the terrible thing you experienced, your mind will subconsciously bring to your remembrance, all your wins, or at least most of them. This will help you to feel better, worry less, and focus on finding solutions for a better life.

BE FLEXIBLE IN YOUR EXPECTATIONS

One major cause of stress is being rigid in your expectations. In your quest to attain a certain position or acquire things, you must give room for uncertainties.

For instance, in the medical practice where you are expected to keep moving up the ladder while writing series of exams to become a consultant, the young doctor may set deadlines such as, "I will be a consultant before 30years of age"

This doctor sets to work. Unfortunately for him, he isn't prepared for uncertainties like failing an exam, strike actions which may delay training, family factors, severe pregnancy symptoms that may delay training, etc.

When such an ambitious individual is met with these unexpected turn of events, he/she may lapse into a period of sadness, which gets worse when they start comparing themselves to colleagues who seem to be moving forward.

This isn't different from the employee who quickly desires a career change, and in his haste, he puts himself under pressure to acquire certain qualifications. This may be a compulsory certification for his dream job. He may give himself some deadlines, but forgets to factor in unforeseeable circumstances such as "not meeting up with the certification within the set time, family factors, etc."

When things don't work out the way he has envisioned it, he gets sad and may even get depressed. This will greatly affect his productivity.

In setting goals, deadlines, ensure they are realistic, ensure you do not already have so much on your table. You must give enough room so that you can combine your present commitments with your goals effectively.

Importantly, ensure your drive isn't borne out of comparison to your colleagues. This is a sure way to stress overload; when you are forcing your legs into another person's shoes without considering their other circumstances.

In the COVID-19 crisis, no one expected the year 2020 to take such a turn.

Imagine setting a major goal that can only be achieved through interaction with people (like event planning, restaurants, etc.), and all of a sudden, you are told to shut down to control the spread of a virus. You never expected it.

How will you feel? Frustrated? Angry? Depressed? These are normal responses, but have you noticed that things happen sometimes for us to explore other more lucrative options, or to pay attention and revive a dying part of our lives, or even to just take a break from the business and pay attention to new growth and development?

Let me tell you what happened to me in 2019.

I had a massive unintentional weight loss due to severe pregnancy symptoms. I lost 10kg to first-trimester pregnancy. It was so bad that I dreaded looking at myself in the mirror or taking pictures.

I remember the day I heard very interesting music. With the little strength I had, I got up to dance. I danced with very low energy, managing to move my body. I decided to do a video recording.

As I saw myself wriggling before the video lens, I almost burst into tears. All I saw was a near skeleton, loosely covered with hanging flesh like that of a frail old woman. My cheeks were grossly sunken with prominent bones everywhere.

I sighed and turned off the video and rather enjoyed the music in peace, besides I was already tired after just 2mins of the dance exercise.

For someone like me, a young lady who never wants to be caught lazy, who sometimes unknowingly takes pride in hard work, who strives to put in her best strength in things that matter, that season of failed strength was enough to drive me into depression.

Here I was spending my 24hours lying down, vomiting frequently with no strength to lift myself. I couldn't read because I noticed I couldn't understand the meaning of sentences.

The worst part is that I entered the year 2019 super-pumped and ready to achieve, with all I had learned from reputable thought leaders about global citizenship. I entered the year with great zeal and expectations to explore and dominate the world.

Now, imagine my helpless self in the first four months of the year unable to do anything and just struggling to get by each day for the sake of the little one growing in me. I couldn't do anything about it.

The situation could have gotten me stressed, how? I had planned on how to go about 2019, but I was limited by my strength.

However, to avoid daily rambling about how my life was over or feeling depressed about things not going as planned or being scared of what the future held and worrying about "wasted months", I quickly applied the last option we talked about in the previous chapter, which is,
"Accepting situations I can do nothing about".

Why "accept"?

I couldn't avoid the pregnancy because it's my child. I couldn't change the situation because it was not a situation I could tell someone to help me reduce the stress.

In addition to that, I intentionally began practicing gratitude for the gift in me instead of focusing on the things I couldn't do.

In other words, you have to accept the fact that some unexpected changes are part of life. Rather than becoming stressed and depressed due to your unmet expectations, be flexible, and remind yourself that it is part of life and keep moving. This will help you cope better and to also identify the reason for the sudden change in season so that you can be better equipped to thrive.

"Some things happen for us to explore other more lucrative options, or to pay attention and revive a dying part of our lives, or even to just take a break from the business and pay attention to new growth and development"

LEARN TO SAY NO

A lot of times, we find it difficult to say no to the other person because we are worried that the person may feel bad. In essence, we accept loads and loads of workload even when it is not convenient. To be in control of stress, you must learn to say NO and also stick firmly by it without being coerced to change your mind.

Someone once replied to my Facebook post, telling me that he had a great opportunity for me.
Well, I had no idea what it was and I directed him to my inbox to talk more about it.

In the course of the discussion, it turned out to be a multi-level marketing (MLM) business with loads of enticing benefits.

For the sake of those that don't know, MLM businesses are business ventures where you get some commission and bonuses as you invite more people to join the company and for using the products of the company.

Who wouldn't want that?

However, I gently declined the offer.

He tried to further persuade me but I remained insistent. As at the time I'm writing this book, I am still building my company, "Healthywealthy Globe".

This means that I can't handle any extra load no matter how enticing or mouthwatering. It will cause me more stress. This is why I emphasize the fact that everyone should know their abilities and capabilities without joining the bandwagon.

You should be able to say NO to friends or family without feeling guilty about it for the sake of your mental health. It does not make you a bad person. It only means that you care well enough for yourself to be able to last and serve people in great health.

But I know that you have a good heart and probably still not sure if you can practice this. Don't worry. I will show you 5 ways to politely decline an offer without any of the parties feeling bad.

Oh dear, I would have loved to help, but......(give your reason)
I'm so sorry, but I'm not in the best position to help right now due to......

I have so much on my table right now, but try contacting……he may be able to help (offer an alternative suggestion)

Thank you for telling me this, but I'm not able to….

If not for…., I would have quickly done it for you

One important thing about using these polite methods is that you have to be resilient enough to stand by your words no matter how much they persist.

SCHEDULE YOUR REST DAY

You see this particular hack, it is a life-saver but unfortunately many don't practice this. We are quick to schedule our businesses, time for clients, time for work, time to learn new things, but the most important part of the schedule is often neglected.

Most people believe that rest is luxury and that is why they use it as a reward for hard work.

However, on the flip side, rest is an essential component of consistent maximum productivity.

Sometime in 2018, I was doing several activities in 24 hours. I had targets but very limited time.

This is an expressway to stress-overload. Because I had set a target for my activities, I was under self-obligation to deliver. I had very good reasons to meet the target as they would affect the course of my life.

I began working back to back. The only time I had to myself was Sundays. However, I still had activities on Sundays, meaning that it wasn't a rest day. Unfortunately, I was performing poorly in the various activities without realizing until my attention was called to it.

I explained why this happened in a concept I created, "THE HEALTHY PRODUCTIVITY CURVE", which you will be learning about soon.

I had to schedule two rest days in a week and there was a remarkable improvement.

What is a rest day?

It is a day you set aside to care for yourself. It can be by sleeping more, getting a pedicure, learning exciting new things, etc. In other words, you are not actively working for others. It is a day you rejuvenate and recharge for a more productive tomorrow.

It is like a car. A day set aside to check the carburetor, paint any scratch, change the oil, and check the tires, etc., so that the car can drive long distances without frustrating you on the road by breaking down.

You get it now?

How do I schedule a rest day?

Choose a day or two days in a week where you declare as self-care or family day, without the interference of any form.

Why should I schedule a rest day?

It spurs your creativity: When you tune off from the focus on so much work, you will realize that you are more relaxed and ideas come best in a relaxed state of mind.

Probably why people get the best ideas while taking a shower.

It gives your body enough time to recover from the wear and tear of previous days.

It prevents overwhelm and burnout.

It helps you work at peak performance. You will be able to perform excellently in all you do.

You will have a reduced risk of depressive moments because you are living a balanced life, without letting any area of your life suffer.

You will become more self-aware. Self-awareness helps you to quickly identify any area of your life that needs fixing before it is too late.

As a creative or one who loves to work, the idea of a rest day can come across as boring. I understand because it was the same for me when I started.

I have compiled this list of things to do on your rest day;

- Meditate and spend quality time with your creator.
- Learn and try out new recipes on YouTube.
- Listen to inspiring messages.

- Get a pedicure or manicure.

- Get a haircut or a new hair-do.

- Read about things to boost your femininity or masculinity or watch others talk about them on YouTube.

- Call family/friends.

- Resist the urge to create content on social media because it will attract comments and make you spend more time replying to them. Remember, it is your rest day.

- Keep a note beside you to jot down ideas you get during this time.

- Learn new exciting things like the culture of some parts of Asia or Africa.

- Binge-watch an interesting TV series that is unrelated to what you do

- Play games.

- Watch funny shows.

- Invest in your non-stressful hobbies. I mentioned non-stressful because a hobby like sewing a sophisticated outfit can be stressful, except you are doing something very simple for the day.

FIND OUT WHAT USUALLY TRIGGERS YOU

Don't skip this. It may sound simple but this is deep. I have had clients who developed some changes in their behaviors, repeated anxiety, due to a stressful situation that occurred a long time ago.

One of my clients who permitted me to share her story experienced serious mental health challenges following an event that happened many years back after delivering her last child.

It was bad that she thought some people were after her life. She visited hospitals several times, spent so much money on tests that were not necessary. The day she understood the root cause of her problems was when she visited a psychiatrist who helped her unburden the troubles of years past.

I will give you another instance. Celia (not her real name) is happily married and has a 2-year old handsome toddler. Recently, Celia observed that she was becoming very resentful. She was easily irritable and nagged at every opportunity. She thought that her new behavior was because of her workplace, however, she wasn't stressed at work. So, Celia decided to be more attentive to situations that set her off.

It wasn't long before she figured it out. She was always triggered whenever her husband showed no interest in helping out with the care of their child. Identifying this trigger helped her address the situation better without wasting time focusing on the wrong thing.

This is to show you that sometimes, we may attribute the cause of our stress to a recent event, whereas it was due to something that happened a long time ago.

Identifying the root cause of your stress can be quite challenging, as you can see from the story of my client who spent a lot before seeing a psychiatrist.

However, this simple exercise will help you.

- Get a pen and paper

- For the next two weeks, note the following:
- The exact moment you feel stressed.
- What triggered it? (an event or a memory)
- How did you react to the situation?
- If you are unable to find a pattern within two weeks, extend it to 4 weeks.

Note that this will require a lot of patience and discipline. In other to help you achieve this, ask yourself; "What is my goal? Why am I doing this?

LIVE IN THE MOMENT

As I write this, we are in the middle of the Coronavirus crisis. I have heard things like, "I can't wait for all these to be over so that I can…" But one thing you don't know is that the more you dwell on the uncertain future, the more you miss all that is happening in the present.

Living in the moment is simply, "MINDFULNESS"

It means that instead of worrying about all you miss and all you are going to do after the crisis, you are simply focusing on how to make the best of the moment.

To further explain mindfulness; when was the last time you stopped to listen to the melodious song from the guitarist playing by the roadside?

Do you know why you did not stop? It is not necessarily because you are chasing after a target or a deadline, but because you did not even notice the guitarist, talk more about considering whether to stop or not.

We live in a fast-paced world where everyone is rushing to catch the train, rushing to work, or school runs, that we have become oblivious to the natural stress relievers around us.

Just observing how the trees sway on a windy day or how humans can conceive great ideas to put up beautiful structures or how beautiful the flowers are, are enough to release happy hormones and help you de-stress greatly.

But these will not happen because while you walk, rather than focus on the moment, your mind is on the food waiting for you at home, the troubles of your kids or even the worries at work, etc.

While it's good to be concerned about these things, however, you will agree with me that worries are unending. Just when you think you are getting a hang of a particular situation, another issue comes up and the worries continue.

So, why not just live in each moment? Be present in activities, and observe factors that make you happy and live healthier and longer. Also, it enhances self-awareness as we described earlier because it helps you notice things that make you feel good or worse so that you can channel your energy much better.

I had a client who had a very challenging family issue. Her major concern that I observed in our discussion was how to reconnect spiritually to God for help. She had attended churches but she felt nothing.

It was obvious that her times in church were not focused on what was going on in the church, but rather her worries, which she quickly agreed to.

I talked to her about being present in the moment, such that if she was in church, she should intentionally focus on what was going on in the church. This helped her to get the maximum benefit from being there.

I must tell you that it is not easy to practice mindfulness when you just begin. You will catch your mind drifting several times from the task at hand.

Because you are on a journey for a better life, intentionally bring your mind back to what you are doing. This will take some conscious efforts and some time. With practice, you will be better at deliberately living in the moment.

PRACTICE MINDFUL EXERCISE

This is also mindfulness just as I talked about earlier, but this time, in addition to exercise. Exercise is beautiful in so many ways: the health of your brain, heart, skin, and virtually every organ of your body.

But do you know that exercise helps you in relieving your stress? I don't mean the rigorous unintentional type like trekking very long distances due to the unavailability of transport. I'm talking about the kind of exercise that helps you release the happy hormones.

For instance, I once had an argument with my friend and it seemed the more we stayed together, the more we had more reasons to argue. My heart was boiling, and I knew that if I continued that way, I may have a troubled mind for a long time.

Quickly, I took an intentional walk exercise to ease the tension. While I walked the streets, I took a mental note of how the cool breeze felt on my skin, I admired the details of the beautiful houses on the street, and I appreciated how colorful everything looked.

I didn't even realize I had done a very long walk and by the time I came back, I was more excited to talk about the things I noticed on the road than to talk about the worries I left behind. I felt so happy, mood boosted and my friend couldn't help but flow in the same excited positive energy I returned with and that was how we ended the argument, in peace and not in pieces.

What I did during that walk was simple. I lived in the moment, focused on the beautiful things of life which lifted my mood and eventually made the initial problem look smaller than I thought it was, even gaining clarity on how to make peace and not prolong the fight.

You can replicate this mindfulness in other activities like swimming, jogging, skipping, dancing, etc.

LISTEN TO UPLIFTING MUSIC

This is one gift to humanity that some people are yet to utilize its full potential. Music is not only for events or special occasions. It is meant to be enjoyed all the time.

Because we are talking about managing stress, the kind of music here is not sad music to make you feel worse about your life, but inspiring music that makes you feel ecstatic.

Have you had that moment when you feel low in energy or unmotivated to work? Play some music and if you can, dance to it. You don't need to know how to dance. Just do things that excite the child in you. These are stress-busters that don't cost anything to harness.

It may not take the worries away but it will help you feel better to eventually find a solution or even to just cope until you can get over it, especially in situations where you can't do anything about it.

As a bonus tip, if you can, listen to the music with an earphone (not too loud and only for a few minutes to avoid hearing damage).

GET QUALITY SLEEP

I'm sure you must have heard things like, "I don't sleep when I am tired; I sleep when I'm done". While this may be a motivational fuel for high fliers, it is an expressway to experiencing the severe consequences of stress such as burnout, depression, and health problems.

Sleep as a stress reliever is a highly productive tool. The reason is that when you sleep, you give your brain enough time to clear off any accumulated toxins from the day's activity.

That is why when you wake up, you feel so refreshed and energized to take on the duties for the day. In essence, if you don't sleep well, the brain gets worked up because you have added extra toxins to the already existing one, giving it more clearing work to do. That is why it gets to a point where your body can't keep up and you just sleep off without warning.

Now, it is not enough to sleep just to check it off your to-do-list. To get the best benefit from sleep, it has to adequate and highly refreshing. This means that you don't need alcohol or any drug to induce sleep and when you wake up, you should not feel tired, headaches, or sleepy during the day. These characterize poor quality of sleep.

Unfortunately, we live in a very busy world where people are made to feel guilty for shutting their eyes even for a moment. That is why you see sleep-deprived people at risk of serious mental health issues. In addition to that, inadequate sleep has been linked to increased risk of a heart attack.

If you must be in control of your stress, you must take your sleep seriously just the same way you will take a medicine prescribed by a physician, because in the true sense of it, sleep is medicinal.

How to get a quality sleep

Some people thrive on 6 hours of sleep, while others require about 8 hours daily to function effectively. This is another reason why you should be self-aware to be able to know how much sleep makes you feel great the next morning. The tips below will help you get quality sleep:

Experiment over the next two weeks on the amount of sleep that energizes you. Note the time you sleep and the time you wake up. This will help you determine how much your body needs. The average rule is 7-8 hours for adults.
Sleep in a cool, dark, and tidy room with minimal or no noise.
Avoid using alcohol or drugs to sleep. If you have sleep problems, consult with a doctor or sleep expert.

EAT HEALTHY FOOD

The only time most people consider being intentional about their feeding habits is when they are on a weight loss journey. However, do you know that there are foods you must eat to combat stress?

If you remember our list of signs of stress-overload, I mentioned eating problems. This means that while some people eat more when stressed, others barely eat anything and both responses have their consequences.

If you eat more, you risk gaining unhealthy weight because of the following:

You have increased craving for sugar and fat.
You don't have time to cook, hence feeding on unhealthy processed foods.

You don't have time to exercise due to the stress.

Also, if you eat less, you are at risk of further reduced immunity, which will increase your risk of getting diseases or difficulty in healing a pre-existing disease. This could be due to;
Reduced appetite for food.
Forgetting to eat.

Now you know how you respond to food when stressed, let's talk about the role of food in managing stress.

Every day, our body is working. Cells are performing one function or the other to keep us going, and as a result, waste products accumulate, which are removed from the body in various ways, like urine, faeces, sweat, etc.

However, there's a kind of waste called free radicals. These "guys" are implicated in several damages, including fast aging, over a long time and the more you work, the more these radicals are released.

But there is good news. The good news is that nature has made it in such a way that most natural foods we eat contain some vitamins to help mop them up. In addition to these, some foods are known to boost your mood while giving you the needed energy when stressed.

What are these natural foods?

Fruits: oranges, watermelons, bananas, etc.

Vegetables: spinach, vegetable pumpkin, celery, etc.

Nuts: walnuts, cashew nuts, peanuts, etc.

Oily fish due to omega 3 contents: salmon, tuna, etc.

Legumes: beans, lentils, chickpeas, etc.

Whole grains: oatmeal, whole wheat, brown rice, etc.

If you noticed, I didn't mention cakes, carbonated sugar drinks, or other processed foods because while these foods will give you a quick burst of energy when stressed, they are not rich in nutrients that will help you combat the damaging effects of stress in your body.

In essence, eat healthy meals not only for weight loss but as a lifestyle for healthy longevity.

MANAGE YOUR TIME

During a stress management workshop I hosted in Qatar, I talked about the importance of managing your time to cope with stress and one of the participants asked me; "I work from 6 am to 7 pm and when I get home, I'm not able to do much again and the cycle continues. It is stressing me. What do I do?"

Quickly, I did a mental calculation to know how many hours he was working. He works for 13 hours out of 24 hours, meaning that he has 11 hours without work. Out of these 11 hours, he may give 1 hour to commuting, 7 hours to sleep, 1-2 hours to eat, and catch up with the news, friends, or any other relaxing activity and then 1-2 hours left. If he was preparing for an exam, he can use 1 hour to read consistently each day.

This practical example is to show you that most times, lack of time is not the problem, but what we do with the time. If you let tiny time-wasters invade your time always, you will always be behind schedule, running late in meeting deadlines, missing out on important life-transforming events due to "not enough time".

Time wasters are real and that is why you may have a job with the deadline in 2 weeks and you waste the first week on them. By the time you enter the deadline week, you become panicky and stressed because you feel you have limited time to meet up to the huge demand.

These time wasters are simple things we may not quickly recognize like social media, television, unnecessary gist time, excessive sleeping, lack of planning, etc.

There are more that are peculiar to us.
Do this simple exercise to identify your time wasters.

Over the next 24 hours, track and record your activities, no matter how insignificant it may seem. This will help you to be accountable for every hour and in no time, you will be more intentional in how you spend your time.

Another way of managing your time to reduce stress is to plan. Don't procrastinate or wait till the last minute before you get things done. Start early.

This helped me when I hosted my first virtual stress management summit. In the two weeks leading to the event, I was so relaxed because I had less to do each day since I had utilized the first two weeks adequately to execute major plans for the summit.

Finally, you must prioritize your activities. Not everything on your to-do-list is important. I attended an event on time management and the speaker told us to think about what we wanted to be in three years. He then asked us to narrow them down to 2 major goals, then prioritize our daily to-do-list to these goals. It means that whatever is on your list that is not aligned to these goals is not a priority.

For instance, you can choose to be a great father and a business owner in three years. That means, your priority for most of your days should be spending quality time with your kids and doing activities surrounding building your business.

UNDERSTAND YOUR UNIQUE PATH

One common stressor that I have observed occurs when you try to compare yourself to another.

You may want to dismiss this because you feel you have arrived at a place of no comparison. Good for you, but you may want to read this first. I gained this insight into owning my unique path after my internship in 2016. Fortunately for me, I ventured into a path that only a few people, especially doctors, are involved in.

As such, I thought I had become immune to comparing myself to another, as I was deeply focused on building my brand.

However, I hosted a successful virtual stress management summit with 6 experts from Nigeria and the UK, as well as 250 registered participants across 6 countries. For someone who was less than 2 years in the stress management industry and yet to grow a team, it was a major feat for me then.

However, I saw an advert of a huge virtual summit by well-known thought leaders. It was huge and had about 3000 registered participants as at the time I registered.

Immediately, I felt bad. I got worked up because I compared my summit with this huge event.

When I felt the negative energy building up, I began asking myself questions like; how can you compare yourself who is less than 2 years in the industry to someone who has been building for many years? Have you forgotten your unique path?

This is the reality of high achievers irrespective of your level in the journey.

If you are starting, you will be tempted to fit your feet in the shoes of someone else doing well. If you are doing well already, you will be tempted to do the same probably for someone with a larger audience.

Understanding your unique path will help you focus on what truly matters without investing in any negative energy from the stress of comparing yourself to another.

The truth is; you don't know their full story, their behind-the-scenes moments, how they started, their sacrifices, etc.

Know your destination and keep your eyes on it without looking left or right, which can be very distracting and stressful.

SEEK HELP

No matter how equipped you are to manage any stress, there are going to be times you feel like you can't continue. There will be times your strength will fail you such that it will be difficult to apply any of the techniques mentioned earlier.

It is very important to recognize this season so that you will seek help quickly. Below are three ways you can ask for help:

Delegate: Listen, you are just one person. No matter how many superpowers you have, if you don't delegate some duties, you will break down quickly or your productivity will drop. This is especially true for online entrepreneurs who are always told to show up for visibility, no matter what. Sincerely, there will be times your health may fail you. Will you still struggle to keep up with the bad state of health? No. Outsource some activities like getting a virtual assistant, hiring a graphic designer, etc.

For the employed, there are going to be times the workload will be more than you can handle. Let me tell you a secret, "if you break down at work, the company will not stop because of you. You will be replaced immediately". I experienced this in my workplace in 2016. I worked excessively trying to impress my "unimpressible" boss. The result was that I broke down.

Immediately, I was replaced until I recovered. If it were in certain workplaces, I will not be paid for the days I was down due to ill health. I once wrote an article on coping with the toxic workplace and I asked, "Are we working to buy illness?" Don't be afraid to speak out when you have reached your breaking point. Request for extra hands, ask for help. You owe it to the people you are responsible for, to be in great health while you earn.

Furthermore, delegating is not only for human resources. You can also employ the services of machines for help such as washing machines to assist you, automating some parts of your business, etc.

Have an accountability partner: To be in total control of your stress, you are going to need an accountability partner. Someone who can look out for you to call you to order when you are going overboard. Sometimes, it is our partners that notice we are stressed due to our incessant complaints, relapse to pre-existing mental health issues, irritability or just noticing that we are working too much. Get yourself someone you trust, respect, and listen to. This is also particularly important for workaholics because after making repeated resolutions to take rest, they tend to relapse over and over into their workaholic lifestyle. If you have a history of mental health challenges like depression, have someone you can confide in and that can check up on you regularly.

Talk to someone (trusted friend, professional, pray): Some stress requires talking to someone for help. It may just be a trusted listening ear or a professional (doctor or psychologist). Talking will help you de-stress a lot and better still help you gain clarity into the problem. In more serious cases like depression, please reach out and get help quickly.

About prayer, some people have wondered the role of religion in managing stress. There have been reports that it is effective. In March 2020, when more countries began recording cases of Coronavirus, google search on prayer skyrocketed. It shows that people were seeking something higher to help them cope with COVID-19 stress. Prayer is a conversation where you pour out your heart and feel calmness afterward because you believe and trust in a higher power (in this case, God) to take care of your worries. I have had clients who tilted our discussion towards seeking God for help. Furthermore, scientists believe that practicing prayer boosts mental health. That means, in addition to the techniques mentioned earlier, practice prayer as a form of spiritual meditation.

CHAPTER 6

Stories Of People Who Successfully Managed A Stressful Situation

To drive home the lessons I have shared so far, I asked some people to send in their stories of how they managed various stressful situations in their lives.

Below are some amazing stories you can learn from.

STORY 1

Sometimes the only way to discover our strength is to go through a period of training that will be stressful.

My name is Ishicheli Grace Kenechi and this is the story of how I built resilience and realized my academic potentials.

As a young girl who grew up in Lagos, Nigeria, I was the only child in a family of 6 children. I had my primary and secondary education in my local area. We were just 5 in my class in primary school and my secondary days as a science student wasn't different as we were just 6 in the class.

I never had a sound academic foundation and this could be because my dad who sponsored my education had only primary school education. My secondary school was not even government approved.

I knew that I wanted more because I felt this vacuum deep within me.

My background wasn't encouraging to the extent that even while I topped the class, my teachers constantly degraded me with the words, "you are just a local champion, and you will realize that you are dull the moment you leave this community. You are a one-eyed man among blind people"

Nothing seemed to be working because my community believed in exam malpractice but I wanted better for myself. I had to work extra hard, reached out to people ahead of me, attended tutorials to pass my high school exam, but all those efforts seemed wasted after our results were seized due to malpractice on the day of Mathematics exam.

I sat for the exam again. This time, I had to overcome the challenge of teachers demanding sex from female students in exchange for answers. Everything was so messed up that by the time our results came out, the English result was canceled as a result of the terrible malpractice in my exam center.

I became frustrated and disappointed that depression set in. I had to encourage myself to try again.

Because I was invested so much in passing English, I passed below average in Chemistry, which was not adequate for my interest in studying Medicine and Surgery.

I did an alternative exam to help me secure an undergraduate degree but it became a disaster due to the change of exam venue without prior notice. I arrived at the new exam venue late and destabilized.

While all these happened, I got enrolled for a diploma in Computer science and eventually began pre-degree studies in Physiology. During this time, I had to retake my high school qualifying exams for the fifth time.

This time, I aced my exams with wonderful grades.

However, I didn't eventually get admission to study medicine and surgery but to study Anatomy, which happened to be my worst choice of study. I cried, asking myself if it was worth all the stress and depression.

But I didn't let it break me and studied relentlessly for my undergraduate degree in Anatomy and today, I am a First Class graduate of Anatomy. I topped my class of over a hundred students, had a CGP of 5.0 five times in 8 semesters and 5 B's in 8 semesters. Maybe I had to write the qualifying exam 5 times too because GRACE is a 5 lettered word and the biblical number for GRACE is 5!!

Stress will strengthen you. No matter how difficult it might be, pick yourself up and take another step in the same direction you once fell.

STORY 2

By Nneoma, Nigerian

My stress started in December 2014 when I got a job at a hotel as a front office supervisor. I was so happy and fulfilled without knowing what was ahead. I was a size 12/14 then.

I took up my responsibilities as a front desk manager. I gave in my best and was noticed and appreciated, which earned me promotions every 6 months. This kept my colleagues wondering and eventually, they got jealous.

I got to the highest position of the Senior Operations manager of a hotel of 136 rooms, with halls of 1200, 200, and 50 people capacity respectively, where meetings and events were held.

I had an extremely strict boss that taught me to take responsibility for everything that happened in the hotel, and I was expected to have figures off by heart in case he calls anytime to get the situation report, which I did with happiness.

I managed the hotel so well that more responsibilities were leveled on me to oversee all departments. I had to leave the hotel at 10 pm, 11 pm, or at midnight most times.

I resorted to eating junk food because I couldn't sit down to plan a healthy meal and eat. I was always on sugary carbonated drinks. I went from being a size 12/14 to size 20/22.

While growing up, I had noticed that stress made me gain weight, feed on junk food, and also forgetful. So, all these symptoms of stress were playing out and I was managing it for 2 years. In 2016, I was accused of falsely and when I was vindicated, I resigned. However, the MD apologized, tore my resignation letter, and asked me not to go. So, I stayed.

The stress continued and my health started deteriorating. My joints hurt, I could not climb my house stairs without panting and my menstrual flow ceased. I was always forgetful and my cholesterol level rose.
Thankfully, an opportunity came again, when I was not appreciated enough for the sacrifices I made for the company.

This time, I resumed work earlier than ever by 6 am, slipped in my resignation letter, and without having another job at hand, I left the company.
They got the letter, the HR pleaded with the MD but this time I decided to take my health seriously by leaving and finding my peace and sanity.

I stayed home for 2 months and rested. I decided to relocate to Lagos for a Visa interview to leave Nigeria but my Visa was denied. Meanwhile while I was home resting, I dropped my CV all over the internet, so I was about leaving Lagos when I was called for a job interview. I was offered the job, I took it.

I had to decide to take my health seriously because I lost my self-esteem. I was overweight because of long-neglected stressors.

I started my weight loss journey by exercising and following a diet religiously and after a year, I gained back my confidence and all I lost to stress, were fully recovered.

My menses flow monthly now, no more joint pains, I climb stairs daily at work (4 story building), I exercise daily, 6 days weekly, I eat clean and healthy and I'm glad I listened to my body and stopped stressing.

STORY 3

By Sana, Indian

Working in the medical profession, work can get hectic. If there's a disease outbreak, our working hours are affected drastically.

One of the most challenging situations that I have had to deal with recently is during one such time at work. As we all know, good medical care involves good teamwork. A team of doctors is involved in examining the patients, others are involved in running special tests and making a diagnosis.

One of my senior colleagues at work was fussy and had a habit of making life difficult for everyone. She usually came late by 1- 2 hours and always gave excuses like doctor's appointments, some work emergency, and not being well.

While we all cooperated with her in every way possible, she started to complain about us to our senior professors to sabotage our work. As the workload increased due to the recent dengue outbreak in my country, we had to stay back till 7-8 in the evening while she ran away by 1 pm.
And despite doing all the work, we would get scolded by our seniors for not working properly.

It got frustrating. I was at work all day and at night, I just complained and whined to my husband and family about how we were being treated at work. After dinner, I would sleep only to wake up and repeat the same cycle of work and complain.

It was particularly challenging as during this time I also had to prepare for an important exam and it was getting impossible. The time was running out and I realized that if I let this affect me, it's only going to steal away from the limited and precious time that I was left with.

I couldn't do anything about her as she was my senior neither could I do anything about the work, so I decided to do something about myself.

I decided to utilize every single minute of my time and began taking my book to work. I started going to work an hour earlier than others so that I could study in peace before other doctors and patients came.

Instead of chatting away in my free time, I chose to study in a quiet corner. Whatever little bit of time I had when I got back home, I utilized it in studying instead of complaining about my day. I started waking up early too so that I could get a good 3- 4hrs of studies before I could go to work.

All of these not only drove me away from the negativity but also gave me a sense of fulfillment as I was able to do justice to my preparation. And after intense hard work, by the Grace of God, I passed the exam with flying colors.

STORY 4

What I do to manage my stress by Vivian, Kenyan.

I make sure I enhance my beauty. I'm not the make-up kind of lady, but I do that when I'm stressed and also use good perfume such that when I look at myself in the mirror, I feel good and forget about the stress.

Another thing I do is to buy something for myself, like a dress, shoe, and perfume just to make me happy.

I'm usually so stressed and sometimes I think too much that I break down, but when I do these things for myself, it uplifts my spirit and helps me appreciate myself more.

Again I listen to loud music and dance for about 30mins.

When I'm thinking too much, I take a walk alone. I change the environment and go by the beach or go on a boat cruise. I may just dress up with my heels, face on point, do my nails, and take myself out for dinner. It can just be to buy a salad of about 5 dollars.

I talk to myself, "Look at this beautiful lady. She doesn't deserve to be going through this kind of stress". This helps me cope better.

Finally, praying and studying my Bible helps me a lot.

SECTION 4

HOW TO BE RESILIENT TO STRESS

CHAPTER 7

Capture Your Thoughts

It is established that your thoughts inspire your actions, which invariably influence your habits. I don't like watching any form of violence or overtly scary incidences unless it is in a movie and I have to remind myself that it is not real. The reason is that, when I watch them, I begin to dream about them and before you know it, I will have a troubled state of mind for a long time, which is not good for me.

Your thoughts are the bedrock of your actions. That is why if you perceive a situation as terrible, it will be terrible and it will influence you to act in a way you may not like in response.

When I taught the members of my Facebook community, Healthywealthy Globe, about "not dwelling on the negatives as a way of managing stress", a member asked me to give him an example. Here is what I told him;

Mr. A and Miss B are in a long-distance relationship.

Miss B reads on social media about how partners always cheat in long-distance relationships.

Following that information, she begins to worry that the worst may happen.

Because she is fixated on a negative outcome in her relationship, she begins to suspect her partner, drawing up conclusions even in things that didn't use to matter. This will put a strain on their communication, which will, in turn, make the lady even more suspicious.

To prevent this, all she needs to do is to avoid such platforms that always paint long-distance relationships bad, focus on the healthy aspects of their relationship, and strive for happiness. She has to learn to avoid dwelling on the negatives which may worsen the situation.

Does this scenario make it clear as to how your thoughts influence your actions and why you should guard your thoughts jealously?

If you want to be resilient to stress, you must filter:

- What your eyes see,
- What your ears hear,
- What your mouth speaks, and
- What your mind thinks.

Stress is how we respond to huge demand or a perceived threat. The word "perceived" means that the situation may not be as bad as our mind thinks it is.

Not long ago, I traveled to the UK without my daughter. The first two nights without her, I worried myself to sleep. I was wondering; "What if she is not lying down well, what if she rolls over on the bed or her head is pressed by something? My mind conceived several negative thoughts because I allowed it, and guess what? I had similar dreams on two consecutive nights. In the dream, her head was badly pressed that I cried till I woke up. I was afraid. I called several times to be sure she was okay and everything was just fine.

After those incidents, I became intentional in capturing my thoughts and refused to dwell on negative thoughts that stressed my life out.

See, if you succeed in intentionally seeing the positives in situations, you have won the greater percentage of your daily battles.

Imagine your child breaking your precious plate. How will you react? You will want to beat her up, right? Now, imagine reminding yourself that she may not have intentionally done that to hurt you. It is also possible that she is not in the habit of breaking plates. So, remind yourself that it is most likely a mistake.

This change in perception is enough to change your disciplinary measure from that of shouting and causing yourself headache; from flogging and building resentment, to that of calmly addressing the situation. This will pass the message that you are not happy with what happened but also that she should be more careful next time to avoid a repeat of the incident.

It begins with your mind.

A simple exercise I want you to do this week is;

No matter what happens, don't react immediately. Take some deep breaths and try to see the positive side of the situation before you respond.

CHAPTER 8

Positive Affirmations

Have you been in a situation where it was obvious that there was a problem, but the assurance that it will be over soon gave you peace of mind?

That is one of the powers of positive affirmation. For instance, during the COVID-19 crisis, we are surrounded by fearful news. You don't know if you are going to be in the next day's statistics, especially if you are going out to work. You don't know if your name is going to be on the next list of retrenched workers. There are so many reasons to be afraid each day and the worst part is that you don't even know when it will all be over.

In moments of uncertainties such as these, positive affirmations are powerful tools because;

- They help you shift focus away from the seemingly unending fears. In other words, it allays your anxieties.
- They help you have a clearer mind to think of the best ways to cope with any unexpected changes.
- They help you build resilience to stress.

Some examples are;

I have clarity of mind to handle this situation.

No one is permitted to pressurize me.

No one is permitted to cause me unbearable stress.

I am thankful for the little things.

This too shall pass.

My mental health is sound.

You can't stress me.

I speak out calmly on things that bother me.

Note that it is not enough to use it just for a day. The more you practice, you build your faith and it becomes a lifestyle, which eventually means greater resilience to stress.

CHAPTER 9

How To Consistently Work At Peak Performance Without Breaking Down

For most creative people, if it is possible, they will like to work round the clock without breaking down or even without sleeping. That is why many have resorted to certain unhealthy habits to keep up, such as binging on coffee, alcohol, smoking, or eating unhealthy food because they don't have time to cook.

That was my story a few years ago. I was one of those who took pride in being a workaholic. For instance, sometime this year 2019, in my last trimester of pregnancy, I took part in two tasking events even though I was not too strong health-wise.

I hosted my first offline class on stress management at 33weeks pregnancy and 39weeks pregnancy, I sat for an exam that spanned for many hours. Even though these were things I could have done after delivery, part of me wanted to feel that sense of accomplishing things that only a few could do when they find themselves in a similar state of health.

In all honesty, while I succeeded in one event, I failed in the other and the reason was quite obvious.

One thing about being a workaholic is that while you may be winning in what you are doing, and getting that fulfillment of getting the job done at all cost, you will also be losing at something else that matters.

It can be your relationship, health, or any other important part of your life. There is truly no pride in being a workaholic.

It is better to practice a balanced work-life and live long and well enough to enjoy the fruits of your labor than to force your body to get everything done at once while other important things suffer.

Most times, we fail to realize the negative effects of such a lifestyle until it gets late.

As I was explaining in a previous chapter, a few years ago before repenting from being a workaholic, I had such a bad experience where I learned the hard way.

It was during a compulsory national program in Nigeria, upon graduation. While I worked, I enrolled in vocational training to acquire the skills of sewing and wig making. While at it, I used the remaining time I had to study and prepare for an exam that would later boost my career.

I ensured that every minute of my life was invested into something productive. As I continued in the super busy lifestyle, it did not occur to me that I was doing myself more harm than good.

When my mum visited me and observed what I was getting myself into, she warned me to take it easy but instead of heeding to her concern, I rather boasted of how I can pull off several activities every 24 hours, less healthy meals, insufficient sleep and lack of rest.

It was not long before my body gave way. I experienced severe weakness and dizziness.

My health deteriorated because I did not take care of it. I was more engrossed in the things I could achieve in a day.

Unfortunately, it was already late because I had to take forceful rest in the hospital. And as expected, my productive days dwindled drastically. It took me time to recover.

To prevent a recurrence, I set aside two days of rest where I will do absolutely nothing related to work, just as I described earlier in scheduling rest days. This intermittent rest has worked for me several times and for some people, I recommended it to.

However, before my health broke down, there were changes in my productivity, which weren't obvious to me. People noticed it and called my attention to it.

In one of the activities I was engaged in then, I was called out for being unserious. In the other activity, where I was learning how to sew, I was always ending up with shabbily-done work.

To me, my 24 hours were occupied, but in the true sense of it, my productivity was a mess.

In this chapter, I am going to use a simple concept, THE HEALTHY PRODUCTIVITY CURVE, to explain to you how you can work CONSISTENTLY at peak performance without breaking down.

THE HEALTHY PRODUCTIVITY CURVE

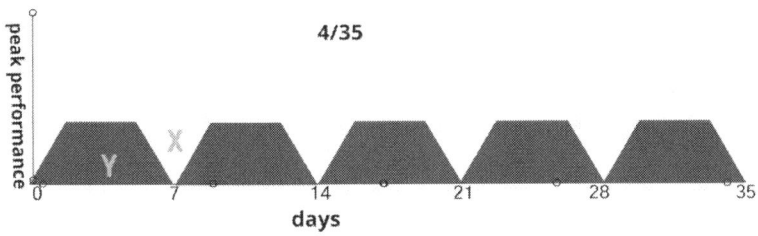

4/35

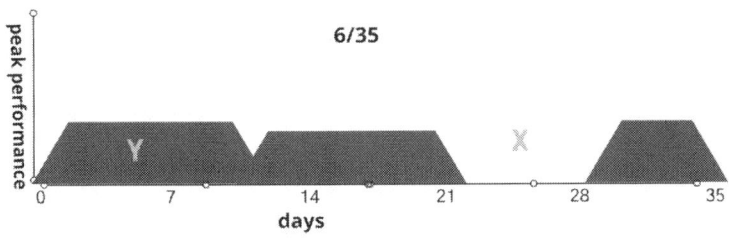

6/35

71

These are curves of two people who worked consistently for 35 days. Th
first curve is Mr. A and the second curve is Mr. B.

X means the period of rest

Y means workdays

FIRST CURVE

Mr. A had a regular pattern of complete rest on the 7th day of every workweek. This means that within the 6 days, he worked at peak performance, yielding the best results. At the end of the 6 days, he rested completely, got back to baseline to rejuvenate so that he could launch out again. He was consistent with this approach of regular intermittent rest for 35 days and at the end of the work period, Mr. A had only lost 4 workdays.

SECOND CURVE

Mr. B started in great spirits to work at peak performance, which he achieved initially. However, he did not schedule any rest day. So, he worked continuously despite his dropping performance. Unfortunately, Mr. B did not even realize that his performance was not optimal as it used to be, because he has not given his body some time to refresh. Eventually, his body could not handle the continuous workload and shut down forcefully.

This made Mr. B take adequate rest (in the worst case, he took the rest in the hospital) for some days for his body to recuperate. He even experienced burnout, which made his recovery time much longer, about 6 days.

By the end of 35 days, he had reduced performance on some workdays, in addition to the 6 days he lost to forceful rest.

Who will you want to be among these two? I'm sure it's Mr. A.

You need to note that the essence here is not just filling our days with work, but working at maximum capacity and seeing results. This is different from just being extremely busy without tangible results.

In other words, to work at peak performance, you must be in great health and include intermittent scheduled rest.

The curve has explained intermittent rest. Other components of great health which you must imbibe are:

Managing your stress

Eating good food

Regular exercising

Getting adequate daily sleep

We have talked about all these in the previous chapters. You don't want to be called the teacher who didn't see tomorrow or the parent who couldn't live long enough to reap the fruits of their labor, or maybe the entrepreneur who didn't last long enough to establish his footprints in the sand of time.

Most people make the mistake of equating happiness to money. In one of my classes, someone said, "The rich don't have any stress. Stress is for the poor" This is a wrong notion. If you are cannot cope with your stress effectively when you don't have, money won't make you any happier.

Before you say I'm wrong, I'll give you instances.

Do you remember the last time you said, "If they increase my salary, I will be among the happiest?" That was my mum's story when she was a teacher. In the early years, she was earned about 2000 Nigerian Naira, which was a huge sum then. She remembered saying to herself, "the day I'll start earning 5 figures as a teacher, I will be very happy"

In her words, "I didn't even realize the eventual increment in my salary to 5 figures because there were extra responsibilities to match the new salary"

Remember those words of Solomon we quoted earlier, "the wiser you are, the more worries you have"

Another instance; Jack Ma, the richest Chinese as at the time this book is written, was asked if he was happier now or when he was a teacher. He replied that he was happier as a teacher than now because just as he is known as the richest Chinese, the same way he is the man with the most responsibilities.

You will agree with me that the more responsibilities, the more stress.
In essence, being able to manage your stress at any point in your life is a necessity. The goal is to live a life of improved health, income, productivity, and happiness. You don't have to wait till you have more money before you pay attention to the other areas. It may just be too late. It is all in your hands. It is either you leave your life to chance or you intentionally make great decisions today that will mostly guarantee you great health, long life, and happiness.

Printed in Poland
by Amazon Fulfillment
Poland Sp. z o.o., Wrocław